Acupressure Points and Massage Treatment

A Practical Guide to Practice Acupressure Correctly at Home to Overcome all common Illnesses and Everything You Need to Know

Dani Twain

Contents

Introduction

The manipulation of acupressure points aims to harmonize the body's energies by stimulating meridians, thereby restoring equilibrium, as balance is fundamental to well-being.

In our modern lifestyle, we've mastered the art of sleeping faster, multitasking meals, and boosting productivity. However, amidst this efficiency, we've lost touch with the concept of balance.

We've all experienced it—whether craving fresh air after prolonged indoor stints or seeking cozy shelter after extended outdoor exposure—our bodies signal when equilibrium is disrupted.

Over 5,000 years ago, the Chinese recognized that applying pressure to specific body areas could alleviate discomfort. Our Western society often instinctively employs this principle, like when massaging shoulder and neck pain.

In this comprehensive guide, we delve into acupressure, exploring its principles, various points, and their therapeutic effects. From enhancing kidney health to alleviating menstrual cramps, migraines, colds, neck stiffness, back pain, fever, and headaches, to aiding weight loss, appetite regulation, digestion, and bolstering positive energy, immune function, childbirth, emotional balance, and illness recovery, acupressure offers a wide array of benefits. Additionally, essential

self-massage techniques for acupressure points are
provided for effective self-care.

Chapter 1

Understanding Acupressure

Acupressure, an ancient healing practice dating back over 6,000 years to traditional Chinese medicine, shares its roots with acupuncture. The term "acupressure" combines the Latin word for needle, "acus," with "press" (premere), while "acupuncture" derives from "punctio" (to prick). Unlike acupuncture, which involves inserting fine needles into specific points on the body, acupressure relies solely on applied pressure.

This massage technique aims to harmonize Qi, the life energy, and restore its flow. In traditional Chinese medicine, disruptions or blockages in the flow of Qi are believed to underlie illnesses and discomfort. Qi travels along meridians, energy pathways throughout the body, where numerous acupressure points are situated. By gently applying pressure to these points, balance in the flow of Qi can be reinstated.

Chapter 2

The Origins of Acupressure

Acupressure, a practice deeply rooted in Chinese medicine, has a rich history centered on alleviating pain, tension, and various ailments that afflict the body. Its core principle involves applying pressure to specific meridian points, aiming to balance the circulation of internal energy associated with physical, mental, emotional, and overall well-being.

While acupressure and acupuncture share common points, the former utilizes manual pressure with hands and fingers instead of needles.

Exploring the Origins

Before delving into historical texts formalizing acupressure, it's vital to recognize the instinctual aspect of massaging pain points. Many of us have instinctively massaged our necks to ease tension or pressed on our temples to alleviate migraines.

This instinctive practice played a pivotal role in the empirical development of acupressure and acupuncture, gradually identifying effective points even before the formalization of meridian maps.

Acupressure emerged as a branch of Chinese medicine, but its earliest documented therapeutic application traces back to an Ayurvedic medicine treatise in India around 5000 years ago. In China, divergent opinions exist regarding its origin, with references to the Tao Yin collection from 2500 years ago. This collection purportedly describes a method of massage or self-massage targeting key points to energize the body and eliminate toxins, laying the foundation for traditional Chinese medicine's expansion across Asia.

The earliest documented reference to the utilization of meridian acupressure points can be traced back to the 2nd century BCE, as acknowledged by archaeologists and numerous historians. This reference, attributed to Sima Qian, recounts the narrative of a Chinese physician defending the therapeutic efficacy of needle and acupuncture practices. Rather than marking the inception of these practices, this account highlights their widespread adoption and official incorporation into traditional medicine.

The historical trajectory of acupressure in China poses challenges for precise delineation, particularly given the Chinese cultural inclination to appraise the effectiveness of practices based on their antiquity. This tendency could potentially inflate the origins of acupressure, albeit of little consequence from a contemporary perspective.

The introduction of acupressure principles to Europe, including France, is credited to a Dutch physician associated with the East

India Company, who allegedly gleaned this knowledge during a sojourn in Japan in 1679. Japan's historical adoption of acupuncture, influenced by its proximity to China and Korea, facilitated the dissemination of these practices.

France's engagement with traditional Chinese medicine, specifically acupressure, commenced notably in the 18th century through publications by Dujardin and Vicq d'Azyr. Louis Berlioz, father of the renowned composer, is purported to be among the earliest individuals to experiment with acupuncture. Despite initial skepticism among medical professionals, interest in these techniques gradually burgeoned.

The burgeoning interest culminated in 1927 with the publication of a comprehensive treatise by George Soulié de Morant, detailing the intricacies of acupuncture and acupressure following his extensive travels in China. Subsequent milestones in France included the establishment of hospital acupuncture consultations in 1932 and the integration of acupuncture into medical procedures covered by social security in 1948.

France emerged as a pioneering nation in legitimizing acupuncture within medical frameworks, exemplified by its inclusion in medical faculty curricula in 1987 and the possibility of acquiring medical qualifications in acupuncture since 2007. Presently, acupuncture practice in France is restricted to physicians, classified not as a specialty but as a recognized medical orientation.

Acupressure, on the other hand, is accessible through various training programs, some of which confer diplomas. Regardless of the modality—whether employing needles or not—the utilization of meridian points remains integral to traditional medicine in China and Taiwan. Hospitals in these regions are renowned for their proficiency in these techniques, attracting patients from across the globe.

Chapter 3

Principles Underlying Acupressure

To grasp the essence of acupressure, it's imperative to delve into the foundational tenets of Chinese and Oriental medicinal practices.

The Doctrine of the Five Elements in Chinese Medicine

Central to traditional Chinese medicine is the doctrine of the five elements:

- Wood
- Fire

- Earth

- Metal

- Water

According to this doctrine, each individual is composed of these elemental forces, with one element typically prevailing. Each element is associated with distinct attributes such as color, significance, emotional state, or seasonal influence.

Yin and Yang: Achieving Equilibrium

Acupressure also hinges on the principles of Yin and Yang, which represent opposing yet harmonizing forces in constant interplay. These forces give rise to Chi, the vital energy essential for balance and well-being.

In Chinese medicine, certain bodily organs are categorized as Yin (e.g., lungs, kidneys, heart), while others are deemed Yang (e.g., stomach, bladder, gallbladder). Imbalances in these forces necessitate diagnosis to identify the underlying causes, enabling targeted acupressure treatment.

Meridians: The Pathways of Vital Energy

At its core, acupressure relies on the concept of meridians, reflecting the holistic interconnectedness of bodily functions according to Oriental medicine.

To maintain Chi's harmonious flow within the body, acupressure leverages the meridian system—a complex network facilitating Chi's circulation throughout the body. These meridians establish connections between internal organs and the surface acupuncture points.

While meridian theory lacks direct parallels in Western medicine, it draws some comparison to familiar systems like the circulatory, lymphatic, nervous, or muscular systems.

According to meridian theory, acupressure targets 12 energy channels, each associated with specific organs:

- Stomach (Yang) and Spleen (Yin)
- Heart (Yin) and Small Intestine (Yang)
- Lungs (Yin) and Large Intestine (Yang)
- Gallbladder (Yang) and Liver (Yin)
- Bladder (Yang) and Kidneys (Yin)
- Pericardium (Yin) and Triple Heater (Yang)

Chapter 4

Benefits of Acupressure

If you're still uncertain about the advantages of acupressure, consider the following compelling reasons that are sure to sway your opinion!

1. Stress and Fatigue Reduction

Acupressure emerges as a potent remedy for alleviating stress and fatigue. This therapy induces relaxation, effectively easing nervous tensions and fostering an overarching sense of well-being. A particularly efficacious acupressure technique involves applying firm pressure to the shoulder point, yielding immediate relaxation.

2. Relief from Aches and Pains

Whether grappling with headaches, migraines, backaches, or toothaches, acupressure proves to be a reliable method for soothing various forms of discomfort. Its efficacy in pain relief stems from two key mechanisms. Firstly, targeted finger pressure on specific points directly soothes inflamed nerves. Secondly, utilizing an acupressure mat triggers the release of endorphins, powerful hormones known for their pain-alleviating properties.

3. Enhancement of Organ Functionality

Acupressure plays a pivotal role in optimizing the functioning of vital organs.

By stimulating these organs, acupressure fosters improved functionality and enhanced release. Targeting specific points, such as those on the right palm and near the wrist, can alleviate heart-related issues and regulate cardiac function, exemplifying the therapeutic potential of acupressure.

Chapter 5

Key Acupressure Points and Their Benefits

Our contemporary way of life, characterized by a frenetic pace, stress, poor posture, and fatigue, exacts a toll on the body, manifesting as tension and discomfort that often go overlooked until they become intolerable.

Common daily afflictions encompass back pain, headaches, neck stiffness, stress, and abdominal discomfort. Acupressure emerges as a swift and effective solution, offering relief and promoting relaxation without the reliance on pharmaceutical interventions.

Lung Meridian Point P7

Situated in the wrist, within a small depression formed when the wrist is flexed, the P7 point of the lung meridian is instrumental in addressing lung and respiratory issues such as asthma, phlegm obstruction, and cough. Additionally, owing to its interconnectedness with the large intestine and synergistic effects with other points, P7 serves to alleviate:

- Headaches
- Neck pain or stiffness
- Psychosis
- Memory problems
- Wrist weakness
- And more

Stomach Meridian Point E36

Positioned along the outer side of the tibia, below the kneecap's mobile part that shifts with foot flexion, E36 serves to invigorate the stomach, fortify the spleen, and regulate blood and Qi circulation. This point aids in treating:

- Stomach-related ailments (vomiting, diarrhea, rumbling, constipation, etc.)

- Mental disorders

- Dizziness

- Stomach pain and ulcers

- Hypertension

- Asthma

- And more

Master Heart Meridian (Pericardium) Point MC6

Located on the lower front, three fingers below the wrist crease, MC6 is highly effective against anxiety and nausea, making it invaluable for managing motion sickness. Its benefits extend to:

- Enhancing blood circulation

- Relaxing the chest

- Alleviating asthma

- Mitigating angina

- Regulating arrhythmia and palpitations

- Reducing stress

- Treating insomnia

- And more

Liver Meridian Point F3

Situated atop the feet, at the juncture between the big toe and the bone of the second toe, point F3 of the liver meridian is instrumental in addressing liver-related issues such as alcohol dependency and the repercussions of excessive or overly rich dietary habits. Additionally, F3 aids in detoxifying the body and offers relief from various ailments including headaches, fatigue, eye inflammation, and bloating.

Large Intestine Meridian Point GI4

GI4 stands out as a frequently utilized acupressure point renowned for its efficacy in alleviating both physical and psychological pain and tension. Positioned on the upper hand, within the cleft formed by the thumb and index finger, this point provides relief from a myriad of conditions including headaches, stress, insomnia, neck or shoulder stiffness, and constipation.

Gallbladder Meridian Point VB20

VB20 boasts numerous benefits owing to its interconnections with other meridians and its proximity to facial nerves. This point proves effective against a wide array of ailments including colds, flu, headaches, dizziness, conjunctivitis, vision problems, deafness, tinnitus, hypertension, epilepsy, insomnia, psychosis, and neck stiffness. Positioned at the neck, beneath the occipital bone at the skull base, VB20 is accessed within the depression formed when the head is inclined forward.

Chapter 6

Effective Techniques for Acupressure Point Massage

Massage of acupressure points diverges slightly from conventional massage practices, adhering to specific guidelines to elicit desired effects.

When targeting an organ for stimulation, massage is conducted counterclockwise, whereas to dampen a bodily function, clockwise massage is employed.

Basic Guidelines:

- Avoid massaging immediately after meals.

- Cultivate a relaxed atmosphere conducive to massage.

- Mild discomfort during massage is acceptable.

Whether utilizing hands or objects like pens, the key is consistent and regular massage of acupressure points to achieve lasting results. Fortunately, the effects are often palpable even after the initial massage session.

A variety of massage techniques cater to different acupressure treatments, tailored to individual preferences and desired outcomes:

1. Strong Continuous Pressure: Applied for 5 seconds to 2 minutes to exert sustained pressure on the point.

2. Beating: Employed by gently tapping or beating the acupressure point.

3. Rubbing: Involves circular or linear rubbing motions over the point.

4. Kneading: Utilized to knead or gently squeeze the point, promoting relaxation and release.

Experiment with these techniques to find the most effective and comfortable method for your acupressure massage regimen.

Chapter 7

Ear Acupressure: Harnessing Reflexology Massage

Ear acupressure stands as a natural alternative modality wherein gentle massage activates various reflex zones within the ear. This holistic approach yields positive effects on both psychological and physical well-being, rendering it a popular practice in both wellness and healthcare domains. Across generations, the intricate structure of the ear and its reflexogenic zones have served as the foundation for therapeutic interventions.

Human Ear: A Multifaceted Sensory Organ with Reflex Zones

Beyond its role in auditory perception, the ear encompasses crucial balance mechanisms and numerous reflex zones. The auditory nerve, along with the inner, outer, and middle ear components, interfaces with the central nervous system to regulate auditory functions. This intricate network collectively constitutes the hearing system, underpinning the ear's multifaceted functionality.

The human ear can be categorized into three main regions:

1. Outer Ear: Primarily responsible for sound reception and coordination.

2.	Middle	Ear:	Facilitates	signal transmission between the outer and inner ear.

3. Inner Ear: Houses the balance organ and translates sound waves into nerve impulses.

Since antiquity, the ear has been recognized as a locus for therapeutic intervention, with various treatment modalities leveraging reflex zones to address diverse ailments naturally. Historical practices, such as bloodletting behind the ear to remedy potency issues in the 18th century, and the use of ear therapy to alleviate back pain dating back to 350 BC, underscore the enduring significance of ear-based interventions in holistic healing approaches.

The reflex zones found in the ear bear resemblance to those present in the hands and feet, forming a sensory map that mirrors the human body's embryonic structure, with the earlobes symbolizing a miniature representation of the head. This anatomical arrangement offers an ideal foundation for alternative healing modalities such as acupuncture or acupressure.

In the realm of traditional Chinese medicine (TCM), records dating back over 2,000 years mention the presence of reflex zones in the ear. The principles underlying alternative practices, including reflex zone therapy, were championed by Fitzgerald, an American physician who initially encountered the technique among indigenous American communities before endeavoring to popularize it across different cultures.

The concept of reflexology massages, pioneered by William Fitzgerald, underscores the intricate interplay between various reflex zones in the feet, hands, and ears, and their connection to internal organs and the nervous system. This connection is facilitated through a network of nerve pathways. In cases of disharmony, palpable tension or hardening may be discerned within the corresponding reflex zone. By applying targeted massage techniques to these trigger points, therapists can elicit beneficial effects that extend to the associated body regions via the relevant channels.

The primary objective of such massages is to address imbalances in a gentle manner. Fitzgerald devised a specialized grid that remains integral to reflexology treatments today. This versatile technique is adept at addressing a wide spectrum of physical and mental symptoms, including pain, tension, or depression, while also fostering localized improvements such as enhanced blood circulation and lymphatic flow. Building upon the principles of reflexology, auricular acupressure emerged as a modern treatment strategy that integrates these fundamental concepts into contemporary therapeutic approaches.

Acupressure Ear: A Modern Approach to Sustainable Therapy

Acupressure ear, categorized within reflex zone therapies, targets bodily ailments by stimulating trigger points located on the ear. These acupressure points represent organs, the nervous system, or serve as reflex zones for pain relief. Rooted in ear acupuncture, often referred to as the "elder sibling" of acupressure, this technique has evolved over centuries, giving rise to various ear massage methods that integrate influences from diverse healing traditions worldwide, including China.

Unlike acupuncture, acupressure entails pressure point stimulation sans needles, employing intensive trigger point massages along with tapping, kneading, or rubbing. This principle aligns closely with reflexology massages, forming an interconnected therapeutic approach.

The common ground between reflexology and ear acupressure lies in their shared efficacy in interacting with the body's systems. Reflexology therapy serves as the foundation for acupressure, furnishing essential insights into trigger points and their connections to organs, joints, and the nervous system—the very essence upon which acupressure hinges.

While reflexology massages typically encompass the entire foot, acupressure confines its therapeutic actions to the ear, thereby streamlining treatment duration and focus. Despite this difference, both modalities exhibit a holistic approach, addressing psychological and physical issues alike.

Echoing principles from traditional Chinese medicine, both acupressure and reflexology leverage the meridian theory, emphasizing the interconnectedness of the central nervous system. Stimulating a trigger point elicits a corresponding response in the associated body part via the intricate network of channels.

Acupressure ear targets specific pressure points on the outer ear, while general reflexology massages encompass all trigger points throughout the body. However, dismissing ear acupressure as less effective or versatile than traditional reflexology would be misguided, as this alternative approach yields multifaceted effects on overall well-being.

The Therapeutic Benefits of Ear Massage: Natural Relief for Diverse Symptoms

Ear massage, incorporating principles of acupressure, aims to restore harmony to the body's meridians, allowing the vital life energy Qi to flow freely and gently addressing both psychological and physical disharmony. Rooted in the teachings of Traditional Chinese Medicine (TCM) and Ayurvedic wisdom, this approach merges ancient knowledge with modern acupressure techniques.

The belief underpinning ear massage is that external influences disrupt the flow of energy, leading to various symptoms. By utilizing ear acupuncture to alleviate blockages, patients experience long-term improvements in their overall well-being. While ear massage shares similarities with acupuncture in addressing functional disorders, it primarily targets minor ailments rather than serious illnesses.

Key areas where ear massage proves beneficial include:

- Pain relief

- Muscle spasms or tension

- Rheumatism

- Hormonal imbalances

- Mental disharmony

- Dizziness

- Lack of motivation and fatigue

- General discomfort

- Toothache

- Lumbago

- Psychosomatic symptoms

- Diarrhea

Ear acupressure is also employed to address addiction issues, offering support for smoking cessation and weight loss efforts. Experienced therapists often utilize ear acupressure points to address multiple symptoms, prioritizing holistic well-being as the ultimate goal.

Despite its numerous positive effects, there are certain conditions for which ear massage is not suitable. These include severe organic problems, inflammatory conditions, or irreparable damage to bones and muscles. Individuals with a weak cardiovascular system should also refrain from this alternative treatment, as stimulation of reflex zones could potentially exacerbate existing issues.

One common criticism associated with acupressure is the tendency for individuals to utilize this gentle procedure as a standalone remedy for symptoms without seeking medical consultation. However, relying solely on acupressure without a thorough examination by a doctor may temporarily alleviate symptoms while masking the underlying seriousness of an existing illness, a scenario best avoided.

It is therefore advisable to consult your physician initially if you experience symptoms, and only proceed with acupressure upon receiving their approval. The latter entails targeting specific acupressure points in the ear as part of the treatment.

Techniques of Ear Acupressure: Diverse Approaches for Vitality

Ear acupuncture points are numerous, each corresponding to different areas of the body. For acupressure to yield optimal results, therapists must possess comprehensive knowledge of each trigger point and its effects.

Six key acupressure points on the ear include:

1. Shoulder and Back Area Trigger Point: Located at the tip of the ear, this point addresses tension, hardness, or pain in the shoulders and back.

2. Organ Reflex Zone: This point is closely linked to all organs of the body, offering relief when stimulated during moments of discomfort.

3. Joint Reflex Zone: With a profound effect on the nervous system, this point alleviates joint pain, necessitating caution and consultation with a physician before treatment.

4. Throat and Paranasal Sinuses Acupuncture Point: Particularly beneficial during or after colds, this point relieves sinus and throat discomfort, promoting relaxation and symptom reduction.

5. Digestive System Trigger Point: Optimal for preventing flatulence or upset stomach, this reflex zone aids in maintaining digestive health.

6. Head and Heart Acupressure Point: Connecting the ear to the head and heart, this pivotal point alleviates headaches and supports heart vitality.

These six reflex zones are arranged in a semicircular fashion along the ear's contour, from the base to the lower lobes. Due to the delicate nature of ear massage, acupressure is often enhanced with aids such as acupressure sticks, ensuring precise treatment of reflex zones and heightened therapeutic efficacy.

Tools for Ear Acupressure: Precision in Targeting Specific Points

Various methods exist to stimulate acupressure points on the ear, with manual ear massage being the most common approach. This technique involves activating all trigger points through a range of pressure techniques. However, alternative options for effective ear acupressure include the use of an acupressure stick, designed specifically for targeting trigger points on the ear.

An acupressure stick, characterized by its narrow design and rounded ball at the end, provides a precise means of treating trigger points on the ear. Available in different diameters and materials such as stainless steel, rose quartz, or wood, therapists should prioritize the quality of the product.

While an acupressure stick enhances precision and intensity in treatment, it is not obligatory for ear massage. However, it can be particularly beneficial for sensitive patients.

Although there may be a misconception that acupressure can be self-administered easily, it is not advisable, especially for individuals with existing medical conditions. Without proper knowledge of trigger points and their effects, attempting acupressure independently may lead to worsened health conditions and ineffective outcomes. Professional training is essential to guide the practical application of auricular acupressure.

Performing Ear Acupressure: Gentle Approach for Deep Relaxation

The process of ear acupressure typically commences with a brief assessment by the therapist to identify hardened reflex zones, which are then targeted for specific treatment. While some therapists utilize specialized devices, others opt for manual palpation of the ear. Once individual deficits are identified, the actual ear massage begins.

The therapist stimulates various trigger points to rebalance the flow of energy, calming or activating reflex zones as needed based on the clinical presentation. Acupressure techniques may include intensive pressure point massage, acupuncture-like needle stimulation, moxibustion for heat stimulus, or a combination of methods. Treatment duration is relatively short, typically lasting a few minutes, with each acupressure point on the ear receiving attention for five seconds to two minutes.

During the massage, patients often experience a pleasant warmth indicative of a therapeutic response. Mild discomfort may arise but usually subsides quickly. Following the session, patients are encouraged to rest, allowing the body to recover from reflex zone stimulation.

Ear acupressure services are offered in wellness practices, by alternative practitioners, in physiotherapy facilities, and even by medical professionals, underscoring its promising potential for the future.

Ear acupressure emerges as a more intensive alternative to reflexology massage, offering gentle relief for both physical and mental imbalances through targeted pressure point stimulation on the ear.

Exploring Acupuncture Meridians

The concept of meridians is a cornerstone of traditional Chinese medicine, where it is believed that the body's life energy, Qi, flows through these pathways. Acupuncture is one method utilized to address any disruptions or blockages in this energy flow, although meridians cannot be anatomically proven by Western medicine.

Meridians and Qi: Foundations of Acupuncture

The human body is traversed by twelve primary meridians and eight secondary ones, extending from head to toe. According to the German Medical Association for Acupuncture (DÄGfA), many of these meridians are named after and associated with specific organs. These organs are further categorized into Yin or Yang, representing feminine or masculine energy in Traditional Chinese Medicine (TCM). While Yang organ meridians typically run along the back or exterior of the body, Yin organ meridians follow paths along the front or interior.

When Qi becomes stagnant within a meridian, it signifies an imbalance of Yin and Yang, which acupuncture seeks to address.

Meridians in Practical Acupuncture

In TCM, meridians not only correspond to specific organs but also various body parts and mental states. Consequently, certain behavioral patterns may indicate physical ailments, a concept not typically associated with Western medicine. For instance, diminished drive or anxious behavior may suggest Qi stagnation in the kidney meridian, according to the DÄGfA.

Acupuncture endeavors to alleviate such blockages by inserting needles at precise points along the affected meridian. By stimulating these acupuncture points, the aim is to restore the flow of Qi and alleviate symptoms. Despite the inability to measure or anatomically verify meridians by Western standards, acupuncture remains an alternative healing practice gaining increasing recognition.

Chapter 8

Acupressure Points for Specific Ailments

Acupressure Point for Headache, Muscle and Bowel Movement

1) Adjacent Valley (Li 4)

Locate the fleshy mound between the base of your thumb and index finger on your left hand. Gently press on this point with your right thumb above and index finger below. Li 4 is renowned for alleviating headaches, easing tense muscles, and promoting healthy bowel movements.

Acupressure Point for Arm Pain and Digestion

2) Pool at the Crook (Li 11)

Position your left arm at a 90-degree angle with the palm facing up. Place your right thumb at the outer end of the elbow crease and apply firm pressure. Li 11, situated at the crook of the elbow, is beneficial for relieving arm, elbow, or shoulder pain and regulating digestion.

Acupressure Point for Skin Problems

3) Sea of Blood (Sp 10)

Sit in a chair with your feet flat on the floor and locate the bulge in your thigh muscles about two thumb widths above the top edge of your knee. Apply firm pressure with your thumbs or the knuckle of your middle finger to the top inside portion of your leg.

Stimulating Sp 10 points aids in purifying the blood and nurturing the skin.

Acupressure Point for Energy
4) Three Mile Foot (St 36)

Identify this point four finger widths below the lower edge of the kneecap and one finger width outside the shinbone. Apply pressure to feel the leg muscle move when flexing your foot. Known for enhancing endurance, especially favored by athletes, stimulating St 36 revitalizes the body's chi, boosting overall energy levels.

Acupressure Point to Relieve Stress
5) Bigger Rushing (Lv 3)

Located on the top of the foot, between the big toe and second toe, find the point by sliding your finger up about half an inch until you feel an indentation. Apply pressure to both feet simultaneously if possible. Renowned as an effective stress-relief point, activating Lv 3 helps alleviate tension and promote relaxation.

Acupressure Point for Sinus Congestion

6) Abundant Splendor (St 40)

Sit comfortably and locate this point halfway between the anklebone and the center of the kneecap on the outside of the leg. Press firmly into the shinbone, then slide your thumb two inches off the bone towards the outside of the leg. Applying pressure here aids in reducing sinus congestion and alleviating mucus buildup.

Acupressure Point for Menstrual Cramps
7) Three Yin Meeting (Sp 6)

Press your thumb into the center of your anklebone, then slide up the inner leg four finger widths. The point is just off the shinbone, towards the back of the leg. Stimulating Sp 6 nourishes energy flow to the spleen, liver, and kidney meridians, making it effective in alleviating menstrual cramps and promoting overall well-being.

Acupressure Points for Kidney Health
8) Supreme Stream (Kd 3)

Locate this point by placing your right thumb on the inside of the prominent bone in the left ankle. Slide your thumb towards the Achilles' tendon, and you'll find the point in the depression between the bone and the tendon. Kd 3 is renowned for its ability to nourish the kidneys, which serve as the foundation of yin and yang energy in the body. Balancing these energies is crucial for maintaining overall health.

Acupressure Point for Migraines, Cold and Neck Stiffness

9) Wind Pool (Gb 20)

Situated along the ridge of the occipital bone and corresponding with the gall bladder meridian, Gb 20 points can be found near the base of the skull. Position your thumbs at the base of your skull near the hairline, then slide them along the bony ridge midway between the spine and the ear. The points lie between the two neck muscles where the neck meets the skull. Applying pressure to Gb 20 can provide relief from tension headaches, migraines, colds, and neck stiffness.

Acupressure Points for Activating the Kidney Meridian

10) Associated Point of Kidney (B 23)

Located bilaterally on the lower back, just above the upper rim of the sacrum, these points are crucial for kidney health. To apply pressure effectively, lie on the floor with a tennis ball positioned under you. For optimal stimulation, use two tennis balls enclosed in a sock to target both points simultaneously. Place the pressure about an inch and a half on each side of the spine. Activating these points stimulates the kidney meridian, which plays a vital role in regulating the body's water flow and maintaining overall balance.

Acupressure Point for Nausea

Which Point? Point PC 6 (Nei Guan or Internal Gate), situated on the inner side of the wrist, 2 cm away from the wrist crease, between the two tendons.

How to Stimulate It? When experiencing nausea, apply firm pressure with your thumb for three minutes. "Do not hesitate to exert strong pressure until you feel a slight tingling sensation," advises Laurent Turlin.

Effects: This pressure point alleviates the diaphragm and harmonizes the stomach. It is particularly effective against nausea in pregnant women, poor digestion, and motion sickness. "The effect is almost immediate. An adult can also easily apply it to a child experiencing car sickness," adds the acupuncturist. Additionally, its stimulation is beneficial for stopping hiccups due to its action on the diaphragm.

Reducing Stress and Anxiety

Which Points? The renowned DM 26 (Ren Zhong or Middle of the Man), located just under the nose, in the middle of the furrow at the upper lip's edge. It can be paired with PC 6 (Nei Guan or Internal Door), situated on the inner side of the wrist, for enhanced effectiveness. For stress and anxiety hindering sleep, use DM 20 at bedtime, also known as the Meeting of the Hundred Vessels, positioned on the skull's top.

Locating the Points: Place the thumbs of both hands above the ears and bring the middle fingers to the skull's midline—the sensitive pressure point is found in a slight depression. Don't overlook C 7 (Shen Men or Door of the Spirit), located at the wrist crease's level, on the outer edge where a small hollow is felt.

How to Stimulate Them? Press on point DM 26 with your thumb for two minutes, directing the movement upwards. "This highly sensitive point may induce a few tears," explains Laurent Turlin. Massage point DM 20 for two minutes just before bedtime.

Effects: Following an emotional upheaval, DM 26 soothes the mind (Shen). DM 20 aids in restoring tranquility before sleep. "Activating it reduces yang, associated with alertness and activity, in contrast to yin, indicative of rest," notes the specialist. C 7 corresponds to the heart's energy, the focal point of emotions. Combining it with PC 6

and DM 20 provides comprehensive relief
for swiftly regaining serenity.

Relieving Back Pain

Which Points? The Ling Gu or Miraculous Bone is situated on the back of the hand, within the hollow between the thumb and index finger. The Da Bai point (Large White) is located at the level of the first phalanx of the index finger, on the outer edge, just before the joint.

How to Stimulate Them? "Massage these two points deeply – don't shy away from some discomfort – one after the other, for two minutes each, while walking to reinvigorate the body's energy," advises the practitioner. Massage the hand opposite the side of the pain. Repeat throughout the day until symptoms subside.

Effects: This effective combination enhances blood circulation, swiftly addressing pain stemming from lower back pain or sciatica.

Lowering Fever

Which Point? GI 11 (Qu Chi, also known as Pond Curve Pond). To locate it, bend your elbow. The point is at the fold's end, towards the outer part of the arm, before reaching the lateral epicondyle of the humerus.

How to Stimulate It? Grasp the elbow with the opposite hand and use the thumb to apply pressure to the acupressure point. Massage firmly in a clockwise direction. Repeat the process on the other elbow as well.

Effects: This point aids in dissipating heat from the body, promoting blood drainage and cooling. It is also utilized to alleviate eczema or hives outbreaks.

Alleviating Headaches

Which Point? Target point GI 4 (He Gu), which corresponds to the fourth point of the small intestine's main meridian. It resides on the outer edge of the index finger, in the middle of the first phalanx.

How to Stimulate It? Massage the entire area of the first phalanx of the index finger on the outer edge for three minutes. "Be cautious, as this point should not be stimulated in pregnant women, as it can induce abortion."

Effects: GI 4 serves as a crucial pain-relief point for the entire body, particularly releasing tension in the face.

Acupressure for Weight Loss

Various studies suggest that regular acupressure practice on specific acupuncture points stimulates the digestive system and facilitates the elimination of excess body fat. This is attributed to the rebalancing of specific energy points.

According to traditional Chinese medicine, the body comprises 12 meridians representing energy pathways. When there are physiological imbalances, this ancient practice posits that the body experiences blockages in these energy channels, leading to slowed internal functions or discomfort.

Efficient digestive function and effective fat elimination are pivotal for achieving a slimmer stomach. However, individuals with excess abdominal fat often struggle with fat elimination and proper digestion.

While dietary adjustments are recommended, their effectiveness can be hindered by a sluggish digestive system and excessive fat storage. Acupressure can play a significant role in eliminating abdominal fat by stimulating specific acupuncture points, thereby enhancing digestive function and regulating appetite.

Given its fat-burning effects, acupressure can complement dietary adjustments to expedite stomach slimming.

Acupuncture Points for Appetite Regulation

If you're new to acupressure, locating acupuncture points on your ear is straightforward. If you struggle with between-meal snacking, targeting these acupuncture points can assist in appetite regulation.

These three acupuncture points can be simultaneously stimulated by applying pressure to the outer part of your ear, situated in front of your ear hole. This area corresponds to where you feel the movement of your jaw under your finger.

As part of acupressure, use your thumb to apply pressure to this area of your ear whenever you experience uncontrollable hunger outside of meal times. Maintain moderate pressure for at least three minutes to experience a reduction in hunger pangs.

Tip: These acupuncture points can also aid in improving digestion post-meal.

GV26 Point for Appetite Suppression

The GV26 acupuncture point, positioned above the mouth, can help reduce appetite. Located between the nose and upper lip, stimulate this acupuncture point by pressing with your index finger on the small hollow between your upper lip and nose. Maintain this pressure for at least five minutes.

Perform this acupressure technique twice daily, ideally between meals when hunger strikes. This practice can assist in regulating your appetite, thereby helping you avoid indulging in sweets outside of meal times.

Enhancing Digestion with the Ren 6 Acupuncture Point

The Ren 6 point offers assistance in improving digestion, effectively preventing bloating or indigestion, which can lead to stomach swelling. To activate this acupuncture point, gently massage the area just below your navel using your index and middle fingers.

Perform this massage for a minimum of two minutes, twice daily. It's advisable to prioritize this acupressure massage after your heaviest meals for optimal digestion support.

Relieving Stomach Discomfort with the ST36 Point

During dietary adjustments, the stomach may experience weakness. To address this, you can stimulate the ST36 acupuncture point, located approximately 5 cm below your kneecap. Note that this point is situated slightly towards the outer part of the leg. To confirm the correct location, move your foot; you should feel the muscle contract beneath your finger.

Apply pressure with your index finger for two minutes. Consistent stimulation of this acupuncture point each day aids in promoting proper food digestion, preventing potential stomach discomfort resulting from gradual dietary changes.

Enhancing Weight Loss with the LI11 Point

Merely adjusting your diet might not suffice to shed excess belly fat. Efficient waste elimination and the reduction of abdominal fat storage demand proper intestinal function. Hence, optimizing intestinal activity is pivotal for achieving a slimmer stomach.

To facilitate this, the LI11 acupuncture point aids in expelling surplus heat and dampness from the body, concurrently enhancing intestinal function.

Positioned at the outer side of the elbow's bend, applying pressure to this acupuncture point for just one minute daily is adequate to enhance intestinal efficiency, consequently fostering belly fat elimination.

Acupressure: Promoting Holistic Well-being

The interplay between body, mind, and emotions forms an intricate trio, wherein each element continuously influences the others. Physical discomfort can impact mental well-being, just as emotions can affect both body and mind. Central to our health and wellness is the concept of balance, which relies on the smooth circulation of vital energy throughout the body via meridians.

When body and mind achieve equilibrium and well-being, we become more adept at adapting to unforeseen circumstances and managing our emotions. Conversely, blockages in the flow of positive energy create an imbalance between the physical and the mental, paving the way for negative emotions, such as stress, and heightening the risk of illness—be it psychological or physical.

Take stress, for example, often triggered by factors like overwork, fatigue, or genetic predisposition. Stress prompts the release of toxins, like excess lactic acid, akin to a sedentary lifestyle or poor blood circulation. This surge in lactic acid promotes muscle fiber contraction, leading to glucose consumption.

This chronic or spasmodic tension keeps the body in a perpetual state of alertness, potentially resulting in various health issues, including heart disorders, sleep disturbances, digestive discomfort, mood disorders, eating disorders, muscle tension or pain, among others. Moreover, stress perpetuates a vicious cycle, making individuals more susceptible to other negative emotions, such as fear, doubt, or low self-esteem.

Acupressure offers a viable approach to stress management by inducing muscle relaxation through pressure application, facilitating the expulsion of toxins like lactic acid, and alleviating psychological symptoms. Acting as a catalyst for well-being, acupressure yields immediate effects, though sustained treatment over several weeks may be necessary to address deep-seated blockages accumulated over time. Its efficacy in promoting relaxation and stress relief has led to its incorporation into health and fitness centers.

Whether administered by a professional or self-practiced, acupressure can serve both therapeutic and preventive purposes. Stimulating specific points—some of which require no specialized technique or training—can aid in holistic well-being. Additionally, acupressure mats, featuring small flexible needles for full-body pressure, offer a convenient means of accessing its benefits from the comfort of home, contributing to emotional health and vitality.

Acupressure: Harnessing Positive Energy

Alternative Chinese medicine modalities, including acupressure, acupuncture, reflexology, and shiatsu massage, operate on a unified energetic framework. According to this concept, individuals comprise Yin and Yang forces, which, despite their opposing nature, harmonize, along with the theory of the five elements—water, fire, earth, metal, and wood—each possessing distinct attributes.

Each element corresponds to specific aspects such as emotions, organs, and seasons. Chinese philosophy recognizes five core emotions: joy, vexation, sadness, fear, and anger. Disruptions in the balance of these forces impede the proper circulation of vital energy through meridians, leading to physical and emotional discomfort.

Emotions, intertwined with organs, have the potential to influence them, manifesting as disorders or illnesses. Conversely, organ imbalances can provoke emotional tensions like irritation, frustration, or anxiety.

Through targeted pressure on specific body points, acupressure alleviates interconnected physical and psychological ailments. This practice fortifies the flow of vital energy, counteracting the circulation of negative energy within the body, thus promoting positive energy and restoring emotional equilibrium in patients.

As a kin to acupuncture, which employs needle insertion, acupressure combats various psychological pathologies. Its utilization in alleviating anxiety, stress, or depression has gained traction, especially in a contemporary landscape characterized by the need for instant gratification and multitasking, compounded by numerous daily demands like work, childcare, household chores, and personal pursuits. Consequently, there is a noticeable rise in patients seeking treatment for emotional concerns during consultations.

In the realm of holistic healing, acupressure emerges as a viable alternative to conventional medications, offering relief from daily blockages. Through targeted pressure on specific points, often forming an "energy bridge," acupressure facilitates the circulation of positive energy, providing a liberating experience by fostering significant emotional release. Notably, the alleviation of negative emotions often correlates with the mitigation or improvement of associated ailments like migraines, sciatica, stomach discomfort, and weight-related issues.

In recent decades, alternative medicine treatments, particularly acupressure, therapeutic massage, and acupuncture, have witnessed widespread adoption. This surge in popularity can be attributed to the rise of modern afflictions and the demonstrable effectiveness of these modalities.

While Western medicine may not fully comprehend the mechanisms behind traditional Chinese medicine, it acknowledges its efficacy. Consequently, acupressure and acupuncture have found application in the healthcare sector, complementing conventional treatments for serious illnesses or pain management, including addressing pain, mitigating drug side effects, promoting relaxation, and enhancing overall mood and well-being.

Enhancing Immunity through Acupressure

In the realm of traditional Chinese medicine, the immune system is conceptualized as Wei Qi, an essential defensive energy circulating throughout the body. This Yang energy serves multifaceted roles, including warming and protecting the body, softening organs, and moisturizing the skin. Wei Qi circulates both on the skin's surface and within the skin, muscles, and organs.

According to traditional Chinese medicine, several organs contribute to the production and dissemination of Wei Qi, including the spleen, lungs, kidneys, intestines, and thymus. Through targeted stimulation of specific acupuncture points, acupressure aids in fortifying these organs and restoring equilibrium to the immune system.

Acupressure, a facet of traditional Chinese medicine akin to acupuncture, shares the same underlying principle of revitalizing Qi circulation by activating the meridians. By addressing energy blockages, acupressure aims to facilitate the restoration of health and well-being.

Distinguishing Between Acupuncture and Acupressure

Acupuncture and acupressure are both techniques rooted in traditional Chinese medicine aimed at revitalizing Qi, the body's vital energy. While acupuncture involves the insertion of fine needles into the skin and tissues to stimulate acupuncture points, acupressure relies solely on finger pressure to achieve the same effect.

One notable advantage of acupuncture is its minimal requirement for equipment, making it accessible and convenient for practitioners.

Acupuncture Points for Strengthening the Immune System

Several acupuncture points are known to bolster the immune system:

- **Stomach 36 (Zu San Li):** Positioned along the stomach meridian, this abdominal master point regulates the spleen, stomach, and intestines, enhancing overall vitality and sustaining health.

- **Kidney 3 (Tai Xi):** Situated between the inner ankle and Achilles tendon, this point regulates Qi circulation in the kidney meridian, fortifying bones, marrow, and tendons.

- **Kidney 27 (Shu Fu):** Located beneath the inner clavicle edge, it relieves lung congestion, alleviates coughs and asthma symptoms.

- **Governing Vessel 14 (Da Zhui):** Found in the upper back at the 7th cervical vertebra level, it acts as a major tonifying point for all Yang meridians, offering relief from fatigue and exhaustion.

- **Large Intestine 4 (He Gu):** Nestled in the fleshy area at the back of the hand between the thumb and index finger, it eases lung issues, alleviates fever, relieves tension, and soothes the mind, serving as a potent pain-relief point and toning the upper body.

During acupressure sessions, the duration of pressure or massage on an acupuncture point varies based on the specific point targeted. However, as a general guideline, applying pressure or massage for 1 to 2 minutes per acupuncture point, once a day, is typically sufficient to promote and maintain health.

It's worth noting that these are just a few examples of acupuncture points among the vast array available for immune system reinforcement. While there are officially 361 acupuncture points, numerous additional points exist, with many situated along the main meridians and others positioned outside these pathways.

Acupressure Point for Childbirth

Once a pregnant woman is acquainted with acupressure, it becomes essential to target reflex zones and pressure points conducive to initiating childbirth and managing labor pains effectively.

The technique remains consistent across all pressure points: using the thumb, gently apply pressure and massage the designated point for one to two minutes with a delicate yet firm touch. The movement can be repeated as necessary based on pain intensity until relief is attained.

Firstly, the most effective pressure point for initiating labor is the fourth point of the large intestine meridian, also known as 4GI, He Gu, or Hoku. Positioned between the thumb and index finger on the hand. To manage contraction pain, stimulating the thirty-second point of the bladder meridian, located in the lower back between the two dimples, is crucial. Additionally, to further stimulate contractions, the twenty-first point of the gallbladder meridian, Jian Jing, situated on the upper back between the shoulder and neck, can be targeted.

While having a certified professional present during childbirth is ideal for precise movement control and extensive knowledge of pressure points associated with maternal pain, acupressure remains an accessible and straightforward practice with numerous benefits. However, caution must be exercised. Seeking medical advice beforehand may be necessary to avoid potential complications related to medical history, especially in cases of intense contraction pain before and during labor.

Therefore, pregnant women, midwives, and partners are encouraged to explore the realm of acupressure for a serene, natural, and pain-free childbirth experience, ushering in the profound joy of welcoming a new life into the world.

Acupressure for Emotional Equilibrium

Merely discussing the physical effects of acupressure in the context of performance enhancement would oversimplify matters and provide an incomplete picture. Why? Because a robust physique alone cannot overcome obstacles without a sufficient dose of motivation and self-assurance, among other factors. Furthermore, emotional equilibrium plays a pivotal role in overall physical well-being, as psychological imbalances often manifest as physical discomfort.

In traditional Chinese medicine, the interconnectedness of the body, mind, and emotions is paramount, with each element intricately influencing the others. Emotions, directly linked to organs through meridians, can disrupt their proper functioning. Hence, the adage "a healthy mind in a healthy body" rings true, underscoring the significance of holistic balance in well-being and health.

When the body and mind are in harmony, emotions remain regulated. However, blockages impeding the free flow of positive energy give rise to restrictive negative energy, permeating the body and exacerbating emotional turmoil. Stress, low self-esteem, anxiety, and fear of failure pose significant hurdles to physical performance.

Acupressure, adept at alleviating bodily tensions and blockages to restore vital equilibrium, facilitates the release of negative emotions, fostering overall well-being crucial for goal attainment. Additionally, it promotes energy production and positive sentiments by inducing relaxation. The pressure applied enables muscle relaxation and toxin release, particularly effective in combating stress, a prevalent malady in contemporary lifestyles. This explains why acupressure complements depression treatment.

Moreover, a healthy body and tranquil mind enhance cognitive faculties such as memory, concentration, and attentiveness.

Acupressure, whether employed to alleviate physical discomfort or restore emotional balance for performance enhancement, can be practiced in various settings:

Under the guidance of a practitioner for therapeutic treatment, especially for physical pain or deep-seated blockages.
In health or fitness facilities for preventive care or relaxation.
At home for daily relaxation and well-being, akin to meditation, utilizing specialized mats or simple self-administered pressure points.
While acupressure is considered unconventional medicine by medical authorities, it's crucial to ensure practitioners have received adequate training in the technique before seeking their services.

Acupressure for a Fit Body

Acupressure offers myriad health benefits crucial for overall performance, exerting positive effects on various bodily ailments. To comprehend its mechanism, one must grasp the tenets of traditional Chinese medicine (TCM) upon which acupressure is founded.

In China and many Southeast Asian nations influenced by Chinese philosophy, medicine adopts a holistic approach, focusing on the individual within their environment. The philosophy revolves around the balance of two fundamental forces:

Yin and Yang, contrasting yet harmonious, akin to magnets with opposing poles;

The five Chinese elements—water, fire, earth, metal, and wood—each associated with emotions, organs, seasons, and animals. From the equilibrium of these forces emerges positive energy. This vital energy, on a human scale, traverses the body via energy channels known as meridians. Meridians are conceptual lines linked to major organs and viscera, and their balance is integral to good health; any imbalance disrupts the circulation of vital energy, leading to physical or psychological ailments.

Acupressure seeks to restore the flow of vital energy by rebalancing the body's energetic forces. Practitioners apply pressure for several minutes on any of the 361 acupressure points identified to stimulate blockages and enhance meridian flow.

Given that the 14 primary meridians extend throughout the body and connect to organs, acupressure alleviates various physical maladies that impede overall performance. Widely utilized in sports, akin to acupuncture—a similar technique employing needles—acupressure addresses:

Muscle soreness post-exercise;

Muscle injuries or trauma;

Tendon inflammation (tendonitis);

Limbs' tension or stiffness;

Rheumatic joint pain;

Sleep disturbances;

Musculotendinous fatigue;

Organic disorders or illnesses (digestive, respiratory, cardiac issues, etc.).

Furthermore, acupressure bolsters the body by promoting swift recovery (muscle regeneration, quality sleep), enhancing physical capabilities (strength, muscle gain, endurance), priming the body for action, and fortifying the immune system.

Using Acupressure to Combat Illness

Apart from bolstering the immune system's production of defenses against pathogens, primarily of viral or bacterial nature, Western physicians have acknowledged the efficacy of employing acupressure to alleviate fever in patients, particularly in cases of severe fever (exceeding 40°C).

When the body confronts an external invader, it triggers its immune defenses, producing molecules called cytokines to alert cells and combat the intruder. Concurrently, the body elevates its temperature to expel the foreign agent. However, excessive fever poses risks to health, prompting the body to dissipate heat through sweating. Applying pressure on acupressure points associated with the gallbladder accelerates fever reduction by facilitating sweating in the patient.

Activating Blood Circulation through Acupressure

Many individuals grapple with blood circulation issues, potentially leading to hypotension (low blood pressure) when venous reflux is impaired. This condition engenders various adverse health effects, including:

Leg discomfort or heaviness;
Dizziness;
Fatigue;
Decreased body temperature;
And more.

By leveraging its ability to stimulate the venous system, acupressure emerges as a remedy against hypotension in high-risk patients, as well as in the management of milder blood circulation ailments.

Utilizing Acupressure for Alleviating Common Aches and Pains

Headaches stand out as one of the most prevalent ailments in France, with three-quarters of adults experiencing them occasionally or regularly, stemming from various causes such as vision or dental issues, illness, fatigue, stress, hypertension, and more. Regardless of the trigger, acupressure proves effective in alleviating headaches, temporal headaches, and migraines. By addressing excessive tension in the cranium, stimulating specific acupressure points can provide relief.

Acupressure for Managing Nausea and Vomiting

In Western medicine, the causes of nausea and/or vomiting are manifold, unlike traditional Chinese medicine, which attributes these symptoms to bodily imbalance (caused by factors like cold, excess heat, or humidity). Associated with the kidney and stomach meridians, pressure points situated along the liver meridian offer relief through acupressure for various conditions such as motion sickness, nausea during early pregnancy, medication-induced vomiting, and more. By restoring the equilibrium of vital forces crucial for good health, acupressure aids in mitigating these discomforts.

Utilizing Acupressure for Alleviating Joint and Muscle Discomfort

Joint and muscle discomfort impacts a significant portion of the population in France, often leading to considerable daily challenges. Stemming from muscle, joint, and tendon dysfunction, these pains frequently manifest as stiffness and discomfort in the limbs.

Employing acupressure for conditions such as rheumatism, arthritis, tendonitis, and musculoskeletal fatigue can effectively diminish pain and discomfort while also mitigating the progression of these conditions by reducing inflammation and enhancing limb flexibility. Notably, both acupressure and acupuncture (using needle

117

pressure) rank among the most effective techniques for managing osteoarthritis.

Acupressure for Alleviating Inner Ear Disorders

The inner ear serves as the body's equilibrium center and movement coordinator, consisting of a small fluid-filled vesicle housing balance receptors activated with head movements. Various health issues can affect the inner ear, including otitis, Ménière's disease, tinnitus, and labyrinth disease.

Traditional Chinese medicine offers remedies to alleviate the symptoms associated with these conditions. Therefore, it is recommended to employ acupressure to alleviate dizziness, nausea, and vomiting induced by inner ear pathologies. This approach is convenient for self-stimulation

of pressure points and yields immediate
results.

Acupressure for Arthritis

The Five Key Points

1. Large Intestine 4

- **Location:** Found in the muscles between the thumb and index finger on the back of the hand.

- **Effect:** Known for its general pain-relieving properties.

2. Gallbladder 34

- **Location:** Situated a finger's width below and in a clear depression in front of the upper head of the fibula on the lower leg.

- **Effect:** Helps alleviate tension in the muscles, particularly effective for musculoskeletal issues.

3. Stomach 36

- **Location:** Best located while sitting, with the hand resting on the kneecap. The point is where the head of the ring finger falls into a depression within the front, lateral shin muscles.

- **Effect:** Supports muscle function, similar to Gallbladder 34.

4. Liver 3

- **Location:** Positioned directly between the foot bones of the big toe and the adjacent toe on the back of the foot.

- **Effect:** Known for its calming properties.

5. Kidney 3

- **Location:** Found at the level of the ankle joint, between the inner ankle and the Achilles tendon.

- **Effect:** Supports joint health according to principles of Chinese medicine.

Acupressure for Managing Childhood Fear and Anxiety

It's common for babies and young children to experience fears, and they may also pick up on anxiety related to special events. However, with simple touches and massages, you can help alleviate your child's restlessness and anxiety. Here's how you can effectively use your hands to massage away fear:

1. Acupressure Point Heart 7 (He 7):
   - **Location:** Ask your child to slightly bend their wrist or hand towards their forearm. The acupressure point is situated on the inside of the wrist, directly on the flexion crease, near the side of the little finger. It can be felt in a depression between two tendons.

- **Technique:** Apply gentle pressure and circular motions for 30 to 60 seconds.

2. Acupressure Point Pericardium 6 (Pe 6):

- **Location:** This point is found on the inside of the forearm, approximately three finger widths away from the wrist crease. It's positioned in the middle between two tendons.

- **Technique:** Use gentle pressure and circular motions for 30 to 60 seconds.

3. Acupressure Point Stomach 36 (Ma 36):

- Location: Instruct your child to bend their knees or legs. The point is located about three thumb widths below the kneecap, approximately one thumb width laterally from the edge of the shinbone towards the outside of the leg.

- **Technique:** Apply firm, vibration-like pressure and circular motions for 30 to 60 seconds.

Tip for Children's Acupressure:

To enhance the effectiveness, lightly massage the following areas on both sides of the body for about 30 seconds each:

- **Forehead:** Gently stroke your thumb from the bridge of the nose (between the eyebrows) towards the hairline.

- **Ears:** Hold the top of your child's ear with your thumb and forefinger, gently pulling the earlobe down.

Acupressure Points for Alleviating Tinnitus

1. Bai Hui (VG20)

- Known as the Meeting of the Hundred, this acupressure point is highly effective in treating tinnitus along with various neurological and emotional disorders. To locate it, visualize a midline drawn above your head (front to back) and a line connecting the tips of your ears. VG20 is situated at the intersection of these lines, between the two parietal holes.

2. Feng Chi (VB20)

- Another potent acupressure point for tinnitus, VB20 also addresses headaches, stiff necks, and numbness. Positioned at the top of the neck, beneath the occipital bone, massage this point by placing your hands on the back of your head and using your thumbs to press towards the inside of your head.

3. Ting Gong (IG19)

- Widely utilized in Chinese medicine to alleviate ear-related issues and calm the mind, Ting Gong is located at the front of the ear, in the hollow in front of the tragus. To find it, open your mouth and feel for the depression at the junction of your jaws.

4. Ting Hui (VB2)

- This acupressure point not only targets tinnitus but also aids in treating hearing loss, itching, toothache, and jaw tension. It can be found just below Ting Gong, approximately a finger's width down.

5. Shuai Gu (VB8)

- Positioned above the ear, VB8 is recommended for addressing damage caused by toxins, such as prolonged analgesic use or antidepressant intake. Locate it two finger widths from the vertical line of the ear.

Maximizing the Benefits of Anti-Tinnitus Acupressure Sessions

To achieve lasting relief from tinnitus, it's essential to massage these acupressure points regularly, integrating them into your self-care routine. While acupressure is effective, it requires consistency for long-term results. Here are some tips to enhance the effectiveness of your sessions:

- Massage points around the ears: Apply firm pressure and perform clockwise massages for 2 minutes.

- Perform back exercises: Lie on your back, flatten your lower back, and bring your knees towards your chest, repeating the movement five times.

- Practice breathing exercises: Engage in Qigong breathing exercises twice daily to counteract tinnitus.

Despite misconceptions, living with tinnitus isn't inevitable. By utilizing the right acupressure points, lasting relief is possible!

Acupressure Points for Alleviating Menstrual Pain

To ease the discomfort of painful periods, here are three acupressure points to target:

1. Sanyinjiao Point: Situated four fingers above the malleolus, this point lies on the inner side of the foot. Apply light pressure and make circular movements for approximately two minutes.

2. Taichong Point: Positioned above the foot, about two fingers below the big toe, this point can be stimulated by continuous pressure, circular massages, or gentle tapping. Experiment with each method to determine the most effective for you.

3. Lower Tian Point: Located three fingers below the navel, this acupressure point can also be massaged, pressed, or tapped to alleviate menstrual discomfort.

Understanding Menstrual Pain in Traditional Chinese Medicine

In traditional Chinese medicine, the balance of the body's energy flow, known as Qi, hinges on the equilibrium of Yin and Yang forces. Any deviation from this balance, such as experiencing menstrual pain, is considered abnormal and indicative of underlying imbalance. Menstrual pain signifies an obstruction in the smooth circulation of energy and blood, rather than a natural or physiological response. It is viewed as a pathological condition, signaling disharmony within the body.

Reducing Menstrual Pain with Acupressure

By stimulating specific acupressure points associated with menstrual discomfort, you can facilitate the body's self-correction mechanisms and promote balance. It is also crucial to adopt a healthy lifestyle, including adequate sleep, nutritious diet, and regular physical activity, to support optimal Qi circulation. Achieving and maintaining balance encompasses both psychological and physiological aspects, necessitating the acknowledgment and management of emotions to prevent strain on the organs. Mental well-being and physical health are intertwined, emphasizing the importance of holistic self-care practices.

Empowered with the knowledge of which acupressure points to activate, you can alleviate menstrual discomfort and experience lasting relief during your periods. Whenever needed, massage the mentioned energy points as frequently as required to manage menstrual pain effectively.

Acupressure Points for Relieving Constipation

1. Valley Union (GI4): Located at the back of the palm, near the base of the thumb, this acupressure point targets constipation. Easily identified by bringing the thumb and index finger together, the protruding flesh indicates the GI4 point. Massage it gently in a circular motion for one to two minutes, up to 4 times daily on each hand. Gradually increase pressure, but if discomfort turns into pain, reduce pressure. Alternatively, tapping can be used instead of massaging.

2. The Ocean of Energy (VC6) and the Pivot Points of the Sky: Positioned beneath the navel, 3 finger widths on each side, VC6 is a potent acupressure point for constipation. It strengthens the large intestine, eases abdominal tension, and promotes digestive tract contractions. Begin by relaxing with deep breaths, then lightly press VC6 with the index, middle, and ring fingers. Hold the pressure for 30 seconds, repeating twice. Massaging in slow, regular motions is also effective.

3. The Winding Pond (GI11): Another effective acupressure point against constipation is GI11. Located at the outer end of the elbow crease when the arm is bent, this point can be stimulated with light pressure in circular motions or gentle tapping using the thumb or index finger. Stimulate both arms for 30 to 40 seconds each, repeating 3 to 4 times daily for constipation relief.

Precautions Before Stimulating These Acupressure Points for Constipation

While these reflex points provide remote stimulation to the intestines, avoid massaging over varicose veins or irritated skin. Individuals with heart conditions, fever, or infectious diseases should consult a qualified acupressure practitioner before stimulation. Pregnant women should refrain from stimulating VC6. Apart from these precautions, regular stimulation of these acupressure points can provide long-term relief from constipation.

Three Additional Practices to Alleviate Constipation Daily

1. Incorporate More Movement:

Combatting constipation requires avoiding a sedentary lifestyle, which exacerbates the condition. Well-oxygenated intestines with toned abdominal muscles facilitate effective contractions. Physical activity also aids in stress management. Alongside acupressure for constipation, aim for at least 30 minutes of walking daily, particularly after meals. Engaging in a weekly enjoyable physical activity like yoga or Tai Chi is also beneficial.

2. Increase Fiber Intake:

Digestion starts in the stomach and proceeds to the small intestine. Remaining food enters the colon, where gradual propulsion to the rectum occurs through regular contractions. To ensure efficient contractions, the colon's food bolus must maintain sufficient volume. Fiber-rich foods, which produce more residue and retain water, help achieve this. Gradually incorporate fiber-rich foods like dried fruits, vegetables, whole-grain pasta and rice, spinach, and bran biscuits into your diet.

3. Practice Morning Qigong Sessions:

In addition to acupressure, Qi Gong, a Chinese energetic gymnastics, can effectively tone the intestines. Here's a simple morning exercise routine:

- Stand with feet hip-width apart, arms at your sides.
- Inhale, pivot your torso and waist on the heel of your left leg, placing your right hand on your stomach and left hand on your kidneys.
- Exhale, bending your torso toward your left leg, allowing your hands to slide over the leg's front and back.

- Hold the position for 30 seconds to 1 minute, then inhale, slowly raising your chest with your head rising last.

- Exhale, returning to the starting position, and repeat the sequence on the right side.

- Repeat each side three times without overexertion.

Acupressure offers effective relief for constipation. Safe and gentle, self-massage and point stimulation can be performed whenever needed. These tips, combined with daily habits, aim to provide lasting relief from constipation.

Acupressure Point And Gastric Reflux

Massage these specific meridians daily for 2 to 3 minutes on each side of the body to significantly alleviate symptoms using acupressure for gastric reflux:

1. VC12: Located between the tip of the sternum and the navel, apply significant pressure to unblock energy.
2. Spleen 4: Found in a small depression between the internal malleolus and the big toe, it harmonizes stomach energy.
3. Stomach 36: Situated in a small hollow one hand's width below the kneecap on the outer edge of the shin, it relieves stomach discomfort.
Additionally, gently massage the entire area beneath the left hypochondrium for gastric

reflux, but be cautious as it may be sensitive during heartburn.

Other Acupressure Points for Enhanced Gastric Health:

For Relieving Bloating:
- Wrist: Target essential points on the wrist to alleviate tension, neck pain, dizziness, and nausea.
- Below the knee: Apply pressure below the knee to ease digestive issues and abdominal discomfort.
- Under the collarbone: Massage this meridian to release tension and promote overall well-being.

For Alleviating Stomach Pain:
The master meridian of the abdomen aids in alleviating ulcers, nausea, and stomach pain.

Located on the outer edge of the leg, 3 finger widths from the kneecap's tip, apply strong pressure using a ping pong ball or your body weight.

To Unclog the Liver:

The detoxification point between the first and second metatarsals aids liver purification and relieves nausea, constipation, and abdominal pain. Massage this area with firm pressure using circular motions for 2 to 3 minutes.

To Reduce Heartburn:

Massage the solar plexus halfway between the sternum and the navel during exhalation to alleviate heartburn, indigestion, and abdominal discomfort. Stimulate the Yuan Qi point, located 2 fingers below the navel, to address digestive issues.

Chapter 10

Four DIY Acupressure Techniques

Acupressure offers the convenience of being accessible anytime and anywhere. While it's not a replacement for medical treatment, especially for serious conditions, it can complement other therapies. Here are some key tips for practicing acupressure on yourself or others:

1. Use your middle finger, supported by your index and ring fingers, to apply firm pressure to the point for two to three

minutes. In some cases, using the thumb or knuckle might be more practical.

2. Sensitivity varies among acupressure points, so adjust the pressure to be strong but not painful. When practicing on someone else, ask for feedback on the pressure, as pain can disrupt energy flow.

3. Apply slow, steady pressure perpendicular to the point, maintaining a 90-degree angle.

4. Gradually apply and release pressure to allow the tissues to respond effectively.